EMPROS MAXIMUS
STAGE 4
FORCED ADAPTATION

The Quick Guide to Professional Level Lifting

Stage 4 - FORCED ADAPTATION
The Quick Guide to Professional Level Lifting.

Why Is This Different –
What The Best Of The Best Don't Tell You

This booklet will be short and to the point. This is not a book on form technique; it is a philosophy of lifting you can use within or to improve a routine. There are plenty of videos on the internet to get form and technique guidance. I will pass on systematized knowledge gained from twenty-five years of lifting with professional body builders, professional power lifters, and Olympic-trainers to up the game in gyms around the world. My hope is that disseminating this information to the average weight-lifter will force professional athletes and coaches to find new and innovative ways to keep the competitive edge, and therefore advance human development to a new level.

Story of experience behind the method – This is a proven systematized workout plan blended together by a curious and experimental mind. This a treasury of mass and strength strategies to supplement and dominate what you have already picked up at the gym or magazines. I had the privilege to lift with the best of the best Pro-Freestyle, Pro-Natural, and Olympic-trainers. I ran my ideas against what I thought could be improvements to their preferred, day-to-day workout plans. My only regret is waiting this long to write it.

This mini manual was written in mind for the beginner as well as the experienced.

Enter at your own risk!

What To Look Forward To – A Case Study

After I experimented (with what you will learn in this short guide) with professionals and average lifters in the gym, it is interesting to see how different genetics and life history respond to this top-level training—but of course, results vary and the heart and drive of the athlete is of top importance, not always genetics, in my experience.

Case Study 1: Male, age twenty-five, 155 lbs. (ending bodyweight 165 lbs., no BMI taken). Never lifted weights. No steroids, no creatine, no glutamine, could only afford one can of protein a month and three small cartons of milk at 10:00 a.m. and 2:00 p.m. Only played baseball in high school. Started this program at age twenty-five and ended a year and a half later.

Starting Bench press: Able to do barbell plus two 10 lbs. plates, six to ten times (65 lbs.). At the end, press 245 lbs., one to three times.

Starting Squat: Squat was 135 lbs. initially, five to six times. At the end, 495 lbs., two to four times, deep, Olympic-squat.

Deadlift: Able to lift 135 lbs. initially, six to eight times. At the end, without practice (about three attempts over the eighteen months), 405 lbs., two to three times. This male was not interested in mass as much as strength. He was not committed to consuming 1.5 grams of protein per body-weight daily.

Case Study 2: Male, age twenty-four, 195 lbs. (ending weight 205 lbs., no BMI taken). Lifted weights since age fifteen. Took creatine, glutamine, and 100 grams of protein powder daily (in addition to 3 regular meals a day), including three small cartons of milk at 10:00 a.m. and 2:00 p.m. on weekdays. Additionally, supplemented with a high-quality men's multivitamin and two to three grams of Vitamin C daily. Played a variety of sports in high school.

Starting Bench press: Able to bench press 315 lbs., two to three times. At the end of one and a half years, press 365 lbs., one to three times (long-term shoulder injury from football prevented progress).

Starting Squat: Squat was 405 lbs. initially, four to six times. At end of one and a half years., press 625 lbs., two to three times.

Deadlift: Able to lift 495 lbs. initially. At the end, 695 lbs., one to two times. This male was interested in mass and was committed to maintaining 1.3–1.5+ grams of protein per body-weight daily.

Preparing For Professional Level Lifting (common sense tips)

Number one: Your body must be prepared to push its limits. No book can guarantee success or prevent injury. You must always consult a doctor, through physicals, as an example, to help you judge whether or not you are healthy enough to lift. Below are some common sense helps for you to checkout:

1) If you are a minor, are you still growing? Doctors can do a variety of things, such as getting an x-ray of your knees, to see if you are done growing. A lifting philosophy of this magnitude can stunt your growth.

2) Are your joints AAA quality? What does this mean? Do you injure easily? Do you twist your ankle easily? If you have lifted before, do your shoulders or knees

hurt when you sleep? Have you snapped an AC joint or torn any ligaments? Have you torn any tendons or muscles, especially in the low back? Any workout program can create injuries anywhere but maxing out your body can reinjure old pain points and create new ones. Make sure you listen to your body. Some of these injuries will re-injure in Stage 4 and cause you to seek restorative surgery.

3) Has your doctor noted that you have a "condition?" Do you have any hereditary issues that may make you prone to high-blood pressure? Atrial Fibrillation? Maxing out your body puts on extreme stress that requires extreme eating and rest.

4) Log all of your max weights for each body part. Take two days, split up the body parts and do one half on day one and then the other half on day two. Make sure to warm up and stretch before maxing out. Do long stretches of thirty seconds or more. Your warm-up should contain at least one to two sets. This will help prevent injury, but this guide will present a very risky way to gain mass and strength.

Critical Mass Philosophy – Setting The Stage

You must warm-up, and you must stretch. This is professional level lifting. Mass is gained primarily in two ways—force the cells to grow with heavy weight or "pump" the cells through repetition or flexing, full of blood, forcing them to grow—forced adaptation.

You must eat like a horse. This is professional level growth. Your body can only absorb so much, and if you overdo it, you can damage organs. Avoid this by consulting your doctor, drink plenty of water, and separate out your meals by at least two and a half hours or as directed by a physician. Any changes in your body or overall health should be noted to your doctor. Some nutritionists note that high-glycemic foods may delay the muscle rebuild process, so therefore, give your body breaks in lifting and eating and avoid refined sugars as much as possible. All the professionals that I have had the pleasure of knowing eventually hate eating. You are probably not eating enough if you love the eating part of your growth.

No repetition (reps) counting (unless wanting to distinguish between high or low rep range)—reach failure on your own, every time. If you are cutting body fat, get a partner and go to beyond failure and allow them to help you with your final reps. Failure Example: You push the bar until you cannot do one more rep; this is failure. Then your partner helps you do a few more reps until you feel your arms fail; this is beyond failure. Excellent for cutting down body fat and enhancing body sculpting.

Don't stop at an arbitrary number of reps. Most professionals are not counting; they are driving the weight until the pain is unbearable. But if you want to track progress with reps, cut the balance between strength and pump—a moderate or medium number of reps per set is five to eight. If you are not feeling extreme pain or pump, you are not achieving a correct mind and muscle connection. Additionally, the five to eight range of reps should set you up to be able to increase the weight a bit, like 2.5 to 10 lbs. per arm or more per leg. Or, you may need to increase the reps for a time and adjust your angles and weight downward until you master the ability to completely fatigue the muscle. Once mastered, go back to upping the weight whenever you are doing a moderate range of reps (five to eight reps, up the weight, repeat). Age, sleep, and quality of food will change your endurance and strength level.

Whole foods are best but harder on the body to digest and less convenient. To get your protein needs per day, you will need to supplement with protein drinks or bars or both.

Maximize each day by paying attention to your body, and it will respond positively. Monitor tendons that are starting to hurt, give them a day or more rest. Monitor soreness—is it Friday and you are still hurting from Monday's bicep workout? You may have a strain, or you are not eating enough to recover. Do you tend to do biceps on day one and then back on day two? This could be the source of over-training your biceps because you are hitting them hard two days in a row. Make sure to separate out your body parts for maximum healing.

Always up the weight for mass and strength, even 2.5 lb. plates are a start. Example: For a particular set, I am doing 60 lbs. on preacher curls. I'll always make sure I do at least 2.5 to 10lbs more on the next set, per side, then repeat that on each set. Always end on your highest weight for muscle memory reasons. In a year, your ending weight today could be your warm-up weight.

Don't get stuck on tracking sets. Shoot for three or four sets per exercise (not body part) but depending on your mood, endurance, music, if you can hit more sets, go for one or two more. Example: You have performed three sets so far on an exercise and not getting the pump or connection you need for growth. Lower the weight, adjust your technique, and try again for another set. If you still cannot achieve a good failure point, then switch to another exercise. If you are getting an excellent pump on a particular exercise at the second or third set, you may want to stick with it for several more sets and go home satisfied.

Number of exercises: You really only need two to three exercises per body part. More can be better, only if you are not getting the pump and muscle failure you are looking for or have plateaued in strength and mass for more than six months.

This technique is done for all body parts. Smaller, denser muscle groupings like calves, biceps, and triceps can take double punishment and respond better to additional reps and sets than other muscle groups—the exception being overloads. Overloads are extremely taxing and can be dangerous if you are not careful and warmed up. Example: Up the number of reps in comparison to other muscle groups for denser muscles. For legs, you might only do two to three reps with heavy weight, yet with calves, you might do ten to twenty reps with moderate weight, upping the weight each time.

START Training!

Before you start, have a listing of all your max personal records for each body part (see back of booklet). Then take these principles and use them for all muscle groups.

Stage 1 - Endurance

Week 1–2

This technique involves reps at a moderate speed, fully under control. Rep this weight as many times as possible. This is to build endurance for the remaining three stages. If you exceed twenty reps, up the weight slightly.

Best to do multiple sets (three to five) and multiple exercises (two to four per body part).

Weight = 25–50% of max.

Stage 2 – Burst Strength

Week 3–4

After two weeks of Stage 1, graduate to Stage 2. Burst is simple, let the weight down/forward slow, and then push or pull with all your strength as fast as possible (do as many reps as possible). With bench-press, for example, bring the weight down slowly, then "burst" the weight up as though you had to throw fire from your chest!

Best to do multiple sets (three to five) and multiple exercises (two to three per body part).

Weight = 44–70% of max. Note: the weight % is increasing.

Stage 3 - Hesitations

Week 5–6

Time to master the weight. Hesitations require patience, strength, and endurance. When any of these three are lacking, you can build them by practicing. During your sets, you will pick either a day to do this with all sets or do it as at first set, progressing to Stage 4 at week 7.

Best to do multiple sets (two to three) and multiple exercises (two to three per body part).

Example: Weight = 40–60% of max. If you are using this as a first set, warm up with this weight at the low range of weight. Next set, proceed to press or pull (depending on the exercise), counting down ten seconds then up ten seconds, or vice-versa, to complete one rep. Do more repetitions till failure. If you were able to do three or more reps, go up to twelve seconds, then fourteen, and so on. Or increase the weight slightly. For example, using bench press, lift-off, slow ten seconds down to the chest, then up slow, taking about ten seconds to the top. Continue till failure (partner recommended).

Stage 4 – Overloads (advanced step) --
Forced Adaptation

**ENTER AT OWN RISK

Week 7–8

Overloads with Olympic-stretching (see below), and then flexing to force blood back into every nook and cranny of your muscles. Best to do with a partner to catch your weight, or on a machine if solo. Make sure your joints are healthy enough to attempt this stage. On week 7, do half your body parts, evenly spread out over the week. On week 8, repeat with the remaining body parts. This is more or less a recovery stage as well as resetting your muscle memory to greater challenges. Do one set per body part unless the max was too easy, then retry by upping the weight slightly.

Question, if you ultimately want to bench 450 lbs., yet you have never attempted 450 lbs., how can you expect to ever get to that weight in a timely fashion? Many times, the pros have simple logic.

Weight ~ 105–110% of max.

Beyond Stage 4

Week 9 – *restart Stage 1–4 cycle, however,* **maintain the Olympic-stretching with flexing on every set, every day, going forward**. Once each cycle has repeated twice (at eighteen weeks), test your max strength on all lifts and update your max charts for each muscle. You should see dramatic increases in your personal records. At this point, update your numbers for overloads to point to your new personal record goals (see chart in back →). If you are not seeing the results, you need to check your daily protein intake typically (and your muscles may need more supplements). Next, check your rest and third, check your drive for domination over the weight, and your muscle pain from the pump or avoidance of it (Not muscle strain or injury. That is a different pain, and you must stop until resolution of the injury). Also, your angles and form may need to be adjusted so that other body parts do not jump in and get worn out before the target muscle gets worn out.

You must use a partner or machine to achieve the overload or risk dropping or pushing the weight away from you. Max out your protein, amino acids, water, and sleep daily. **Note:** Pull exercises with overloads is a risky and difficult task. It requires extreme health and some creativity if you do not have a partner. This philosophy is easier for push exercises but pull exercises benefit as well. Take deadlifts for example, you would need to rest your barbell in a Smith Cage like you were going to do shrugs. Then shrug the weight up, then deadlift it down, very carefully, beyond your max weight, to the floor. Or take bicep curls as another example. A partner would be required to get the weight up, then you would take the weight down in a slow and controlled manner, and then drop it. Lat pulls would be the opposite. You would need a partner to pull the weight down with you, and you would let the weight up very slowly, keeping your legs pinned under the knee bar so you don't go up with the bar off the ground. Again, this puts extreme stress on your tendons and muscles. Pull exercises put your body more open to injury than push due to the nature of the body mechanics. You could still use this philosophy of lifting to failure, flexing, stretching, and then upping the weight to increase mass and strength dramatically over traditional methods.

Key #1 Olympic-Stretching – Beyond Stage 4

Olympic-stretching is the edge professionals don't typically reveal. Do this with every set going forward from now on.

Muscle hooks: Forcing your muscles to max capacity means forcing all of your muscle fibers to fire. Olympiads like to stretch constantly to make this happen. Some will stretch muscles for one to three minutes to have advantages over amateur athletes, prior to working out. Others stretch thirty seconds between sets to max out all the available strength. The **difference** is when you stretch, push/pull hard against the object to achieve an extreme stretch. For example, when stretching one side of your back (latissimus dorsi) and holding onto a fixed object, hold to stretch your back muscle (as you normally do), **then pull towards you at the same time you stretch, as though you are doing a repetition for your back muscle! Normally, you just hold and stretch, but this new way is like one long repetition after your set.** Make sure the object you use to stretch is stationary (does not move). This maxes your capacity for strength over time. It feels like you are doing a rep for that muscle group, and to an extent, you are. Your body will be forced to adapt to the new condition. Then, flex your muscle as hard as you can for a short period of time (five to twenty seconds). This will max out your capacity.

Key #2 Protein Intake – Mixed Proteins

Muscle magazines have it right. Approximately 80% of gains are attributed to eating, not lifting, once the right workout is performed.

Mixed Protein Sources: These greatly magnify the amount of nitrogen in the system. In fact, in your blood, you want to prolong the nitrogen level as this signifies your recovery period. In the last couple decades, a lot of study has gone into this science, and protein provider companies have followed suit with new protein blends. Do your research.

Protein Amount: Nutrition science has told us that just to maintain muscle, you need approximately one gram of protein per body weight pound. Meaning, if you are 200 lbs. and you hit the weights today at a moderate to extreme level, you need 200 grams of protein the next twenty-four to forty-eight hours during the rebuild stage. If you lift the next day and only get 150 grams of protein in the first twenty-four hours, you are looking to get 250 grams of protein in the next twenty-four to forty-eight hours just to maintain muscle. You want to go beyond this intake, in the example above, to ~250 grams of protein (200*1.25) or more for mass building. Of course, the previous muscle needs starts to diminish, but new lifting days begin the next cycle of requirements. Thus, you can see why eating is the main vehicle to growth. Most professionals will tell you that eating is the key priority over gym time, otherwise, you will cannibalize your repairs from other muscle groups.

Protein Timing: The breakdown of food into the needed recovery elements occurs right away in your bloodstream and remain there approximately four hours, according to research. Best to eat every three to four hours (during the day) to maintain nitrogen levels for recovery, however, do your research in regards to what triggers insulin. If your insulin is elevated all the time, you will have heath repercussions down the road and sabotage your gains. To drastically reduce waste in the body and further enhance your gains, supplement branched-chain amino acids as well as L-glutamine with each meal.

Key #3 Supplementation

Best bang for your buck: Creatine, L-Glutamine, and Multi-vitamins.

Creatine: Start slow and see how your body metabolizes it. Best to get substances that have multiple pathways into the system, i.e. various forms such as alkaline creatine, phosphorus creatine, and the like.

Glutamine: Take a heaping teaspoon when you wake up, with each meal, and when you go to bed. Glutamine is the primary amino acid in your muscle. When you take it at this frequency, you maximize the number of proteins created by your body, thus minimizing aminos going into the toilet and increasing your mass and recovery. As discussed above, get products that have multiple forms of glutamine, such as phosphoric or alkaline glutamine if able.

Multi-vitamins: Best to get an expensive men's/women's supplement from well-known brands in your local vitamin shop. Take them regularly when lifting; back off when taking breaks.

Multi-vitamins/Supplements in general: Purchase high-quality products. Don't purchase cheap products. Consult the local vitamin seller for the best quality for your money. If you add creatine and glutamine and other aminos, high-bioavailable nutrients are best for absorption. Example: Fermented aminos or creatine with forms that have more than just mono-hydrates.

Eat freshly squeezed lemons and limes in the AM with your amino drinks for faster recovery and alkaline your body. Supplement your recovery with buffered vitamin c and astaxanthin.

Testosterone Boosters: Pick natural boosters for long-term growth and to stay in the game as an athlete. If you cut corners and pick the synthetic things, you will have joint consequences, mood swings, and expensive Post-Cycle Therapies.

Drugs: If you are not going to listen to the experts on avoiding performance enhancing drugs, read the book *Death in the Locker Room, by Bob Goldman,* to get more information on the warnings and nutrition needed to support drugs in your system.

Wisdom Note #1 - Cutting Weight

The "six-pack" comes from time in the gym and eating correctly. Cut out small things such as cooking oil, bread, or dairy that can cause bloating and digestive stress. Foods that are low on the glycemic index must be priority. Otherwise, the insulin boost may force the body to store fat.

If cutting weight, do the multi-set style of lifting to failure (you can't do another rep) and beyond failure (you can't do another rep even with partner helping you with the weight) before eating in the morning using super-sets with no rest (circuit training) for extreme fat burning.

Wisdom Note #2 - Pain and Soreness Are Your Preachers; Listen To Them

If the muscles are sore to the touch for more than twenty-four to forty-eight hours, you may have a muscle strain, or your protein intake may be too low. Doing overloads would be an exception. Muscle soreness for a week is normal at times if you are going extra heavy on the weights (such as, you found a good muscle connection with several sets, was feeling super strong, had no distractions, adrenaline music in the ears, and pre-work out chemicals in the system).

Tendon pain: Make sure you stay on top of this and give this program a rest until you get to the bottom of pain that may be attributed to a tendon. Tendons can undergo small tears that only get worse if you do not rest and reduce inflammation. This path of ignorance puts many professional athletes back six months or more due to surgery rehabilitation. Do the rehabilitation first, lower the weight dramatically, and wait till the pain subsides! Listen to your doctors and physical therapists.

Devastating Mix to Avoid Plateaus

Some of my experiments involved mixing up these stages in one day or for mixed days in a week to keep the muscles from plateauing, as well as keeping it fun and challenging. For example, set one, after warm-ups, do the endurance Stage 1 with lots of reps. For the second set, do the burst Stage 2. Thirdly, set 3 is hesitations, and then try a max or overload Stage 4 set, all the while doing the Olympic-stretching and flexing between each set. Stage 4 at this point will be difficult, but that is the beauty of the challenge. A partner is highly recommended.

We pull it all together!

Week 1

Day One Example Chest:

Stage 1 - Endurance

(3X sets plus warmup) Bench Press (with partner preferred): Your max is 250 lbs. Warm up with 100 lbs. (40% X 250 lbs.). Let the weight down reasonably fast and press with the same speed up. The main goal is to get as many reps as possible, but do not go too fast as that is reckless and you could get an injury. If you exceed twenty reps, up the weight.

(3X sets plus warmup) Chest fly, machine, or dumbbells. Your max on dumbbell press is 160. Warm up with ~40% of your max (30 lb. dumbbells = 60 lbs.). Do as many repetitions as possible. If you exceed twenty reps, go up to 35 lb. dumbbells.

(3X sets no warmup) Chest press with dumbbells. Your max on dumbbell press is 160. Warm up with ~40% of your max (30 lb. dumbbells = 60 lbs.). Do as many repetitions as possible. If you exceed twenty reps, go up to 35 lb. dumbbells. If you exceed twenty reps again, go up to 40 lb. dumbbells and so on.

Fast-forward

Week 3

Day One Example Chest:

Stage 2 - Burst Strength

(3X sets plus warmup) Bench Press (with partner preferred): Your max is 250 lbs. Warm up with 150 lbs. (60% X 250 lbs.). Let the weight down in a slow and controlled manner and press up fast with all your strength. The main goal is to envision the need to throw something heavy off of you, from your chest. This stresses the muscle in more of a "fight or flight" scenario, causing muscle memory and growth. If you exceed ten reps, up the weight approximately five to ten lbs. per arm. Repeat or change the beginning max percentage, up or down based on your performance. Your goal is to keep going up in weight.

(3X sets plus warmup) Chest fly, machine, or dumbbells. Your max on dumbbell press is 160. Warm up with ~40% of your max (30 lb. dumbbells = 60 lbs.). Do as many burst repetitions as possible. If you exceed fifteen reps, go up to 35 lb. dumbbells.

(3X sets no warmup) Chest press with dumbbells. Your max on press is 160. Warm up with ~40% of your max (30 lb. dumbbells = 60 lbs.). Do as many burst repetitions as possible. If you exceed fifteen reps, go up to 35 lb. dumbbells. If you exceed fifteen reps again, go up to 40 lb. dumbbells and so on.

Fast-forward

Week 5

Day One Example Chest:

Stage 3 - Hesitations

(3X sets plus warmup) Bench Press (with partner preferred): Your max is 250 lbs. Warm up with 100 lbs. = 40% of max. Let the weight down very slow and controlled. Take at least ten seconds to go down then press up with the same speed, take ten or more seconds. If you exceed five reps, up the weight approximately 5–10 lbs. per arm. Repeat or change the beginning max percentage, up or down based on your performance. Your goal is to keep going up in weight.

(3X sets plus warmup) Chest fly, machine, or dumbbells. Your max on dumbbell press is 160. Start with ~40% of your max (30 lb. dumbbells = 60 lbs.). Again, count to ten as you go down slowly, then count to ten again as you go up, ending at the top with ten seconds.

(3X sets no warmup) Pick another chest exercise and repeat the above.

Fast-forward

Week 7

Day One Example Chest:

Stage 4 - Overloads with Olympic-stretching

(1 set plus 2X warmup) Bench Press (with partner preferred): Your max is 250 lbs. Warm up with 100 lbs. = 40% of max, do a few repetitions, do regular stretching. Then warm up with 200 lbs.—one rep—stretch and rest. Overload 265 lbs. =105% of max (250X1.05~262). Let the weight down at a moderate to slow speed. Attempt to press it up. If you cannot, let it fall carefully (under a machine bar as an example) or let your partner take it up for you. If you get any out of the ordinary pain, stop immediately, and wait till next time. When complete, grab an object to stretch your chest. Pull hard against the object like you are trying to move the object with your chest. Do this for ten to thirty seconds. When completed, flex your chest as hard as you can for ten to thirty seconds. Record your weight attempted and if the set was completed, up your new personal record and if able, attempt the weight again if you feel good.

Thank You For Reading!

This is your map to extreme growth. Replicate these principles for each body part, doing overloads with exercises you are comfortable with and those that you want improvement on, such as triceps press for triceps, preacher curl for bicep, and so on. If you are noticing less improvement on one body part or exercise, arrange your schedule so you can start the week with that exercise.

From here on, do your Olympic-stretching and flexing on every set going forward, all the while, trying to increase the weight on **each set**:

Mass and Strength Summary

1) Lift till failure
2) Flex
3) Olympic-stretching
4) Up the weight
5) Moderate rest 30 seconds to two minutes, two to four minutes for leg day
6) Finish multiple sets and change exercise.

Cutting Body Fat

1) Lift till failure
2) Flex
3) Olympic-stretching
4) Cut the weight 20–80%;
5) Lift again with little or no rest
6) Repeat
7) Finish multiple sets and change exercise.

Devastating Mix Challenge

1) Stage 1 till failure

2) Flex

3) Olympic-stretching

4) Stage 2 till failure

5) Flex

6) Olympic-stretching

7) Stage 3 till failure

8) Flex

9) Olympic-stretching

10) Stage 4 modified—max or exceed max

11) Flex

12) Olympic-stretching

13) Repeat on new exercise.

Progress Chart And Max Calculations On Next Page →

Max Progress Chart

	Max #1	Max #2	Max #3	Max #4	Max #5
Presses					
Barbell Bench Press					
Dumbell Chest Press					
Shoulder Press					
Squats					
Pulls _(extreme caution when attempting pull Overloads, partner or machine required)_					
Dumbell Curls					
Lat Pulls					
Shrugs					
Deadlift					

CalC Chart

Max weight x Max % = Training Weights for each Stage

		40% Max	60% Max	105% Max	107% Max	110% Max
Presses						
Barbell Bench Press						
Dumbell Chest Press						
Shoulder Press						
Squats						
Pulls (extreme caution when attempting pull Overloads, partner or machine required)						
Dumbell Curls						
Lat Pulls						
Shrugs						
Deadlift						

Progress Chart - examples	Date___	Date___	Date___	Date___	Date___
Barbell Bench Press					
Dumbell Chest Flys					
Dumbell Chest Press					
Shoulder Flys					
Shoulder Press					
Preacher Curls					
Dumbell Curls					
Tricep Press					
Leg Curls					
Leg Extension					
Leg Press					
Squats					
Deadlift					
Lat Pulls					
Rows					
Lateral raises					
Shrugs					

Max Progress Chart

	Max #1	Max #2	Max #3	Max #4	Max #5
Presses					
Barbell Bench Press					
Dumbell Chest Press					
Shoulder Press					
Squats					
Pulls *(extreme caution when attempting pull Overloads, partner or machine required)*					
Dumbell Curls					
Lat Pulls					
Shrugs					
Deadlift					

CalC Chart

Max weight x Max % = Training Weights for each Stage

	40% Max	60% Max	105% Max	107% Max	110% Max
Presses					
Barbell Bench Press					
Dumbell Chest Press					
Shoulder Press					
Squats					
Pulls (extreme caution when attempting pull Overloads, partner or machine required)					
Dumbell Curls					
Lat Pulls					
Shrugs					
Deadlift					

Progress Chart - examples	Date___	Date___	Date___	Date___	Date___
Barbell Bench Press					
Dumbell Chest Flys					
Dumbell Chest Press					
Shoulder Flys					
Shoulder Press					
Preacher Curls					
Dumbell Curls					
Tricep Press					
Leg Curls					
Leg Extension					
Leg Press					
Squats					
Deadlift					
Lat Pulls					
Rows					
Lateral raises					
Shrugs					

Progress Chart	Date___	Date___	Date___	Date___	Date___

Progress Chart	Date____	Date____	Date____	Date____	Date____

Progress Chart	Date____	Date____	Date____	Date____	Date____

Progress Chart	Date____	Date____	Date____	Date____	Date____

Progress Chart	Date___	Date___	Date___	Date___	Date___

Progress Chart	Date____	Date____	Date____	Date____	Date____

Progress Chart	Date____	Date____	Date____	Date____	Date____

Progress Chart	Date___	Date___	Date___	Date___	Date___

Progress Chart	Date____	Date____	Date____	Date____	Date____

https://store.bookbaby.com/book/Stage-4-Forced-Adaptation

Print ISBN: 978-1-66780-445-3 (softcover)
eBook ISBN: 978-1-66780-446-0 (eBook)

This is the First Edition of Stage 4 – Forced Adaptation 2021.